MW01519169

Easy Diabetes Cookbook Perfect for Beginners

Start Cooking Simple and Healthy Meals

Evelin Turk

Table of Contents

Almond Cookies

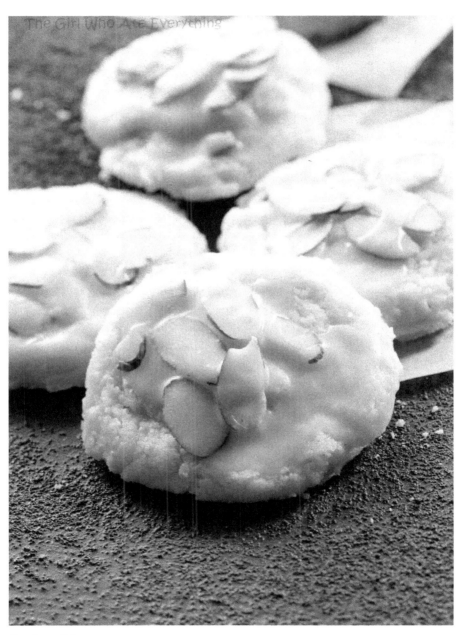

Servings: 24

Ingredients:

1 cup slivered almonds

1/2 cup (1 stick) unsalted butter, softened

1/3 cup confectioners' sugar

1 large egg yolk

1/2 teaspoon almond extract

1 cup unbleached all-purpose flour

1/4 teaspoon salt

24 whole almonds

Directions:

1. Place the slivered almonds in a food processor and process until finely ground.

2. Place the butter in a large bowl and beat at medium speed with an electric mixer until fluffy. Gradually beat in the sugar. Beat in the egg yolk and almond extract.

3. Add the flour, the ground almonds, and salt and beat at low speed just until blended. Cover and refrigerate until chilled, about 2 hours.

4. Preheat the oven to 325°F. Line 2 baking sheets with parchment paper.

5. Shape 24 level tablespoonfuls of the dough into balls. Place 1 1/2 inches apart onto the prepared baking sheets. Place a whole almond in the center of each ball, pressing to flatten the dough slightly.

6. Bake until the bottoms of the cookies are lightly browned, about 15 minutes. Cool on baking sheets 2 minutes. Transfer to racks to cool completely. Store in an airtight container at room temperature for up to 3 days.

Nutrition Info:

7 g carb, 94 cal, 7 g fat, 3 g sat fat, 19 mg chol, 1 g fib, 2 g pro, 25 mg sod • Carb choices: 1/2; Exchanges: 1/2 carb, 1 fat

Tapenade

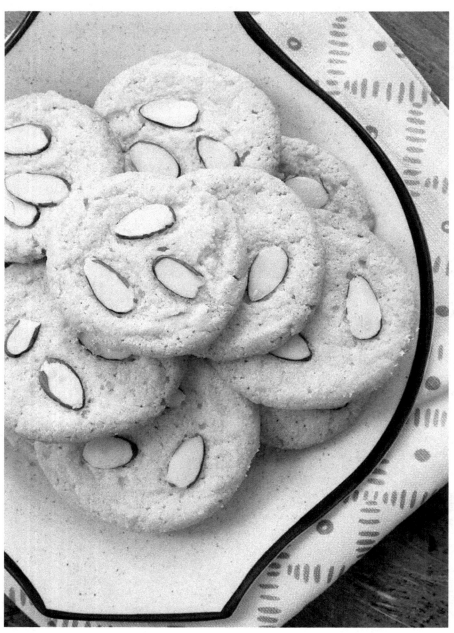

Servings: 1/2 Cup

Ingredients:

1/2 cup niçoise olives, pitted

2 tablespoons chopped fresh Italian parsley

1 tablespoon capers, rinsed and drained

2 canned anchovy fillets, drained

2 teaspoons grated lemon zest

2 teaspoons lemon juice

1 small garlic clove, minced

1/8 teaspoon freshly ground pepper

2 tablespoons extra virgin olive oil

Directions:

1. Combine all the ingredients except the oil in a food processor and pulse until finely chopped. Add the oil and pulse to combine. The tapenade can be refrigerated, covered, for up to a week.

Nutrition Info:

1 g carb, 58 cal, 6 g fat, 1 g sat fat, 1 mg chol, 0 g fib, 0 g pro, 206 mg sod • Carb Choices: 0; Exchanges: 1 fat

Farro And Vegetable Risotto

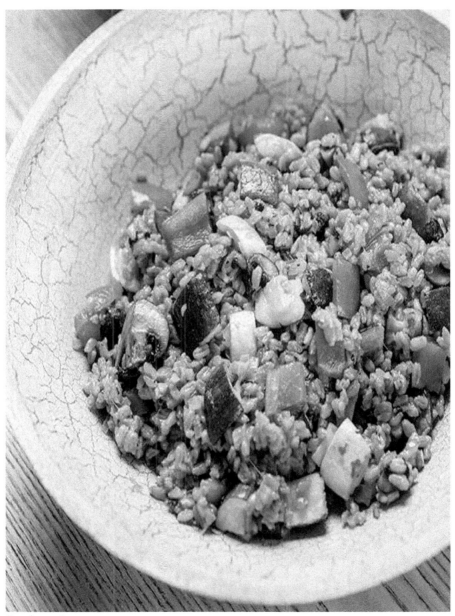

Servings: 8

Ingredients:

4 cups Vegetable Stock or low-sodium vegetable broth

2 teaspoons extra virgin olive oil

8 ounces sliced mushrooms, any variety

1 small onion, diced

1 cup farro

1/2 teaspoon kosher salt

8 ounces asparagus, tough stems removed and spears cut into 1 1/2-inch pieces

2 packed cups chopped fresh spinach

2 ounces freshly grated Parmesan (about 1/2 cup)

1/8 teaspoon freshly ground pepper

Directions:

1. Pour the stock into a medium saucepan and bring to a simmer over medium-high heat. Reduce the heat to low and keep the stock warm.

2. Heat a large saucepan over medium heat. Add the oil, mushrooms, and onion and cook, stirring often, until the vegetables are softened, 8 minutes.

3. Add the farro and salt and cook, stirring constantly, 2 minutes. Add the stock, 1/2 cup at a time, stirring frequently, until the liquid is absorbed after each addition before adding more broth. After 30 minutes, stir in the asparagus and continue adding broth and stirring until the farro is tender, about 5 minutes longer. Stir in the spinach and cook, stirring constantly, until the spinach is wilted, about 1 minute. Remove the saucepan from the heat and stir in the Parmesan and pepper Spoon the farro into a serving dish and serve at once.

Nutrition Info:

17 g carb, 125 cal, 3 g fat, 1 g sat fat, 4 mg chol, 3 g fib, 6 g pro, 225 mg sod • Carb Choices: 1; Exchanges: 1 starch, 1/2 fat

Italian Turkey Meatloaf

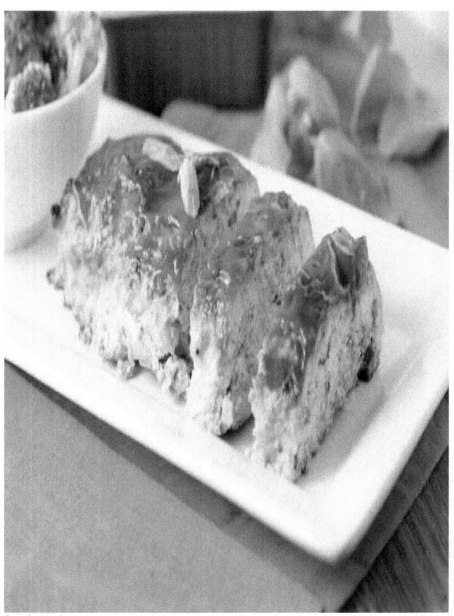

Servings: 6

Ingredients:

8 ounces white mushrooms

2 teaspoons extra virgin olive oil

1/2 cup finely diced onion

1 garlic clove, minced

1/2 teaspoon kosher salt

1/2 teaspoon dried oregano

1/2 teaspoon dried basil

1/4 teaspoon freshly ground pepper

1 pound ground lean turkey

8 ounces Italian turkey sausage, casings removed

3/4 cup no-salt-added tomato sauce, divided

1/2 cup plain dry breadcrumbs

1/3 cup 1% low-fat milk

1 large egg, lightly beaten

1/4 cup chopped fresh Italian parsley

Directions:

1. Preheat the oven to 350°F.

2. Place the mushrooms in a food processor and pulse until finely chopped.

3. Heat a medium nonstick skillet over medium-high heat. Add the oil and tilt the pan to coat the bottom evenly. Add the mushrooms and onion and cook, stirring often, until the vegetables are softened and most of the liquid has evaporated, 8 minutes. Add the garlic, salt, oregano, basil, and pepper and cook, stirring constantly, until fragrant, 30 seconds. Transfer to a plate and let cool slightly.

4. Combine the turkey, turkey sausage, 1/4 cup of the tomato sauce, the breadcrumbs, milk, egg, parsley, and the mushroom mixture in a large bowl. Mix thoroughly with your hands. Place the mixture in a large shallow baking dish and shape into a 10 x 4-inch loaf.

5. Spread the remaining 1/2 cup tomato sauce over the loaf and bake 1 hour. Let stand 5 minutes before slicing. Cut the meatloaf into 6 slices and serve at once.

Nutrition Info:

13 g carb, 218 cal, 10 g fat, 2 g sat fat, 85 mg chol, 1 g fib, 20 g pro, 411 mg sod • Carb Choices: 1; Exchanges: 1/2 starch, 1 veg, 2 lean protein, 1 fat

Thin-sliced Green Beans with Pine Nuts And Mint

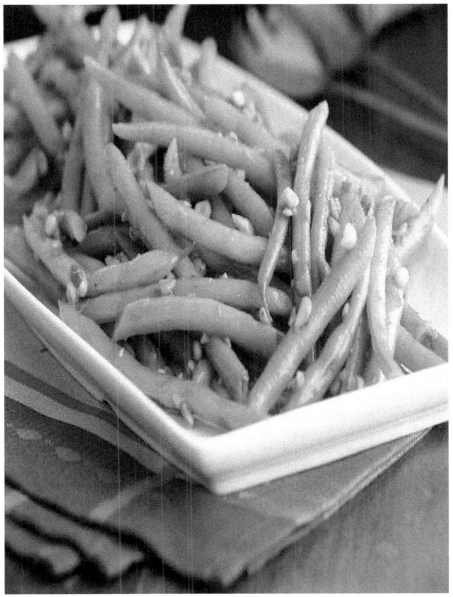

Servings: 4

Ingredients:

2 teaspoons extra virgin olive oil

1-pound green beans, trimmed and cut on the diagonal into 1/2-inch slices

1/2 teaspoon kosher salt

2 tablespoons pine nuts, toasted

2 teaspoons chopped fresh mint or 1 tablespoon chopped fresh basil or Italian parsley

Pinch of freshly ground pepper

Directions:

1. Heat a medium nonstick skillet over medium-high heat. Add the oil and tilt the pan to coat the bottom evenly

2. Add the green beans and salt and cook, stirring constantly, until the beans are crisp-tender, about 4 minutes. (If you like beans more tender, add 2 tablespoons water, cover, and cook an additional 1 to 2 minutes.) Remove from the heat and stir in the pine nuts, mint, and pepper. Spoon the green beans into a serving dish and serve hot or warm.

Nutrition Info:

8 g carb, 81 cal, 5 g fat, 1 g sat fat, 0 mg chol, 4 g fib, 2 g pro, 146 mg sod • Carb Choices: 1/2; Exchanges: 1 veg, 1 fat

Cranberry-orange Pancakes

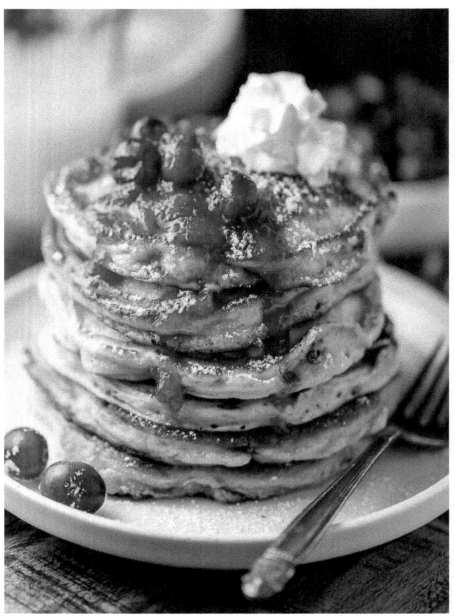

Servings: 6

Ingredients:

2 navel oranges

3/4 cup unbleached all-purpose flour

3/4 cup whole wheat flour

1 tablespoon sugar

2 teaspoons baking powder

1/4 teaspoon ground cinnamon

Pinch of salt

1 1/4 cups plain low-fat yogurt

1 large egg

1 tablespoon plus 1 1/2 teaspoons canola oil, divided

1 teaspoon vanilla extract

3/4 cup fresh cranberries or unthawed frozen cranberries

Directions:

1. Preheat the oven to 250°F. Place a large baking sheet in the oven.

2. Remove 1/2 teaspoon of the zest from 1 of the oranges and reserve. Cut a thin slice from the top and bottom of the orange, exposing the flesh. Stand the orange upright, and using a sharp knife, thickly cut off the peel, following the contour of the fruit and removing all the white pith and membrane. Holding the orange over a bowl, carefully cut along both sides of each section to free it from the membrane. Discard any seeds and let the sections fall into the bowl. Drain the orange segments, reserving 1/2 cup of the juice. Reserve any remaining juice for another use. Repeat with the remaining orange.

3. Combine the flours, sugar, baking powder, cinnamon, and salt in a large bowl and stir to mix well. Combine the yogurt, orange juice and zest, egg, 1 tablespoon of the oil, and the vanilla in a medium bowl and whisk until smooth. Add the yogurt mixture to the flour mixture and stir until a smooth batter forms.

4. Heat a large nonstick griddle or large nonstick skillet over medium heat. Brush with 1/2 teaspoon of the oil using a silicone brush. Spoon the batter by scant 1/4 cup measures onto the griddle 4 at a time. Sprinkle about 1 tablespoon of the cranberries onto each pancake. Turn the pancakes when the tops are covered with bubbles and the edges look cooked. Place the pancakes on the baking sheet in the oven to keep warm. Repeat the procedure with the remaining oil, batter, and cranberries to make 12 pancakes.

5. Place 2 pancakes on each plate. Using a slotted spoon, top each serving of the pancakes with about 1/3 cup of the orange segments.

Nutrition Info:

45 g carb, 258 cal, 5 g fat, 1 g sat fat, 39 mg chol, 4 g fib, 8 g pro, 215 mg sod •
Carb Choices: 3; Exchanges: 2 starch, 1/2 carb, 1/2 fruit, 1 fat

Steak with Quick Mushroom-rosemary Sauce

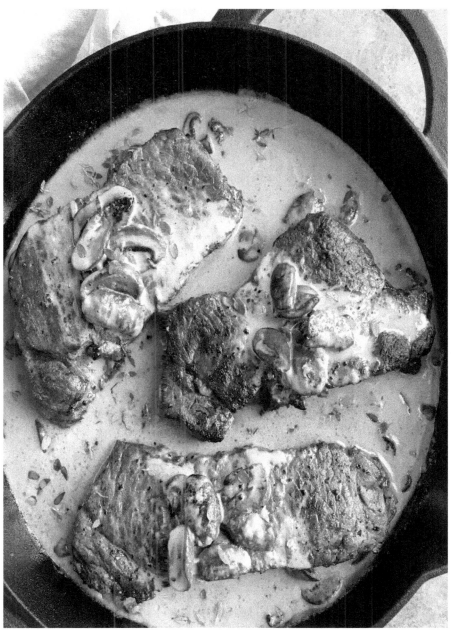

Servings: 4

Ingredients:

1 (1-pound) strip, top sirloin, tri-tip, flank, or ranch steak, trimmed of all visible fat

3/4 teaspoon kosher salt, divided

1/4 teaspoon plus 1/8 teaspoon freshly ground pepper, divided

4 teaspoons extra virgin olive oil, divided

2 garlic cloves, minced

8 ounces cremini or white mushrooms, thinly sliced

1 large tomato, chopped

1/2 cup dry red wine

2 teaspoons chopped fresh rosemary or 1/2 teaspoon dried rosemary, crumbled

Directions:

1. Sprinkle the steak with 1/2 teaspoon of the salt and 1/4 teaspoon of the pepper. Heat a large heavy-bottomed skillet over medium-high heat. Add 2 teaspoons of the oil and tilt the pan to coat the bottom evenly. Add the steak and cook, turning once, 4 minutes on each side, or to the desired degree of doneness. Transfer the steak to a cutting board, cover loosely with foil, and let stand while you make the sauce

2. Add the remaining 2 teaspoons oil to the skillet and tilt the pan to coat the bottom evenly. Add the garlic and cook, stirring constantly, until fragrant, 30 seconds. Add the mushrooms, tomato, wine, and rosemary and cook, stirring often, until the mushrooms are tender and most of the liquid has evaporated, 6 to 8 minutes. Stir in the remaining 1/4 teaspoon salt and remaining 1/8 teaspoon pepper.

3. Cut the steak across the grain into thin slices and divide among 4 plates. Top with the mushroom sauce and serve at once.

Nutrition Info:

4 g carb, 228 cal, 9 g fat, 2 g sat fat, 42 mg chol, 0 g fib, 26 g pro, 266 mg sod • Carb Choices: 0; Exchanges: 3 lean protein, 1 fat

Carrot And Orange Puree

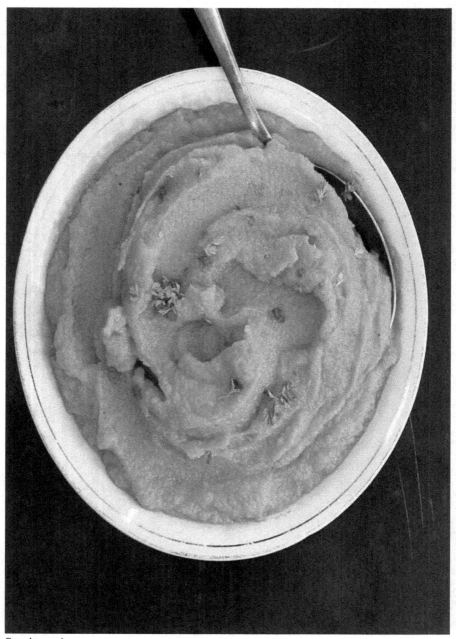

Servings: 4

Ingredients:

1-pound carrots, peeled and sliced

1 cup orange juice

2 garlic cloves, sliced

1 small navel orange

2 teaspoons unsalted butter

Pinch of kosher salt

Directions:

1. Combine the carrots, orange juice, and garlic in a medium saucepan. Bring to a boil over high heat. Reduce the heat to medium, cover, and cook until the carrots are very tender, 20 to 25 minutes. Drain the carrots in a colander, reserving the cooking liquid.

2. Meanwhile, remove 1/2 teaspoon of zest from the orange and reserve. Cut a thin slice from the top and bottom of the orange, exposing the flesh. Stand the orange upright, and using a sharp knife, thickly cut off the peel, following the contour of the fruit and removing all the white pith and membrane.

3. Holding the orange over a bowl, carefully cut along both sides of each section to free it from the membrane. Discard any seeds and let the sections fall into the bowl.

4. Place the carrot mixture, the orange segments, orange zest, butter, and salt in a food processor. Process until smooth, adding the reserved cooking liquid a few teaspoons at a time, if needed, to reach a smooth consistency. Spoon the carrots into a serving bowl and serve hot or warm.

Nutrition Info:

19 g carb, 96 cal, 2 g fat, 1 g sat fat, 5 mg chol, 3 g fib, 2 g pro, 88 mg sod • Carb Choices: 1; Exchanges: 1/2 fruit, 2 veg, 1/2 fat

Lemon-basil Shrimp with Linguini

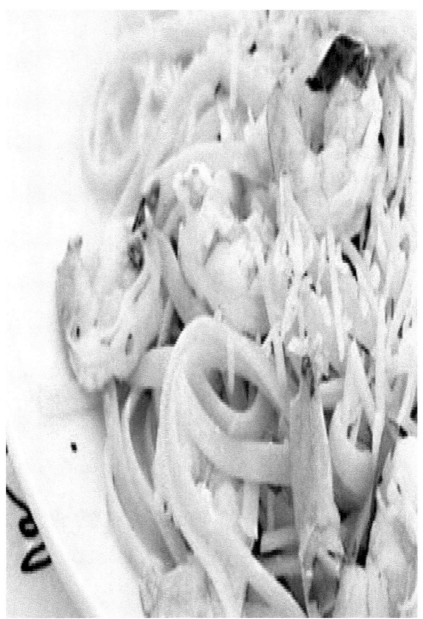

Servings: 4

Ingredients:

1 (9-ounce) package fresh whole wheat linguini

2 teaspoons extra virgin olive oil

1 small onion, halved lengthwise and thinly sliced

2 garlic cloves, minced

1/2 cup dry white wine

1/4 teaspoon kosher salt

1/8 teaspoon freshly ground pepper

1-pound medium peeled deveined shrimp

2 teaspoons grated lemon zest

2 tablespoons lemon juice

2 tablespoons chopped fresh basil

Directions:

1. Cook the linguini according to the package directions.

2. Meanwhile, heat a large nonstick skillet over medium-high heat. Add the oil and tilt the pan to coat the bottom evenly. Add the onion and cook, stirring often, until softened, 5 minutes. Add the garlic and cook, stirring constantly, until fragrant, 30 seconds. Add the wine, salt, and pepper and bring to a boil. Cook until the wine is reduced by half, about 2 minutes.

3. Add the shrimp and cook, stirring constantly, just until the shrimp turn pink, about 2 minutes. Remove from the heat and stir in the lemon zest, lemon juice, and basil.

4. Divide the linguini among 4 plates and top evenly with the shrimp.

Nutrition Info:

34 g carb, 322 cal, 6 g fat, 1 g sat fat, 206 mg chol, 5 g fib, 28 g pro, 452 mg sod • Carb Choices: 2; Exchanges: 2 starch, 3 lean protein, 1/2 fat

Grilled Artichokes with Olive Oil And Lemon

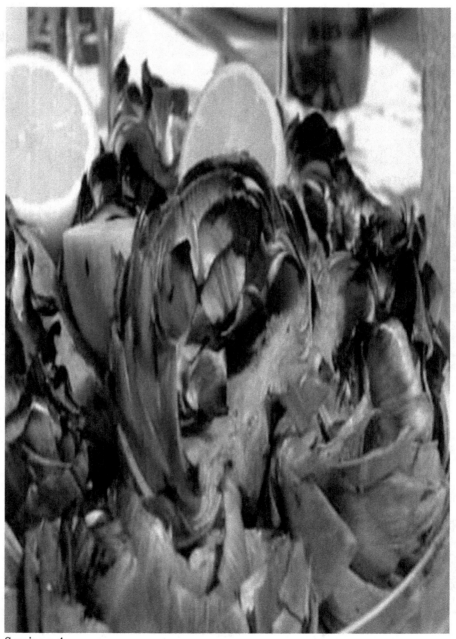

Servings: 4

Ingredients:

4 medium artichokes

2 teaspoons plus 1 tablespoon extra virgin olive oil, divided

3 tablespoons lemon juice

1/2 teaspoon kosher salt

Directions:

1. Place the artichokes in a large pot and add water to cover. Bring to a boil over high heat, reduce the heat, cover, and simmer until just tender when pierced with a knife, 35 to 45 minutes. Drain the artichokes and let stand until cool enough to handle. Cut each one in half lengthwise and remove the fuzzy center choke using a spoon or a melon baller.

2. Prepare the grill or heat a large grill pan over medium-high heat.

3. Brush the artichokes with 2 teaspoons of the oil. Grill, turning occasionally, until the artichokes are well browned and very tender, about 15 minutes. Place the artichokes in a serving dish.

4. Whisk together the remaining 1 tablespoon oil, the lemon juice, and salt in a small bowl. Drizzle the mixture over the artichokes and serve hot or at room temperature.

Nutrition Info:

14 g carb, 115 cal, 6 g fat, 1 g sat fat, 0 mg chol, 7 g fib, 4 g pro, 254 mg sod • Carb Choices: 1; Exchanges: 2 veg, 1 fat

Blueberry–poppy Seed Coffee Cake

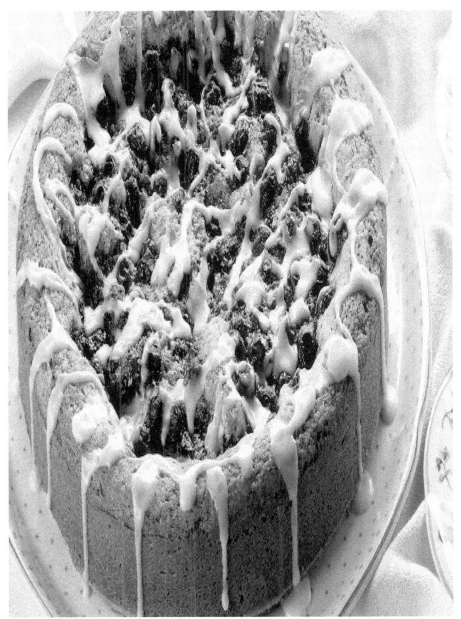

Servings: 16

Ingredients:

1 teaspoon plus 1/4 cup canola oil, divided

1 cup whole wheat flour

3/4 cup sugar

1/2 cup unbleached all-purpose flour

1 tablespoon poppy seeds

1 teaspoon baking powder

1/2 teaspoon baking soda

1/4 teaspoon salt

3/4 cup low-fat buttermilk

1 large egg

1 teaspoon vanilla extract

2 teaspoons grated orange zest

1 cup fresh blueberries or unthawed frozen unsweetened blueberries

Directions:

1. Preheat the oven to 350°F. Line the bottom of an 8-inch round cake pan with parchment paper. Brush the side of the pan with 1 teaspoon of the oil.

2. Combine the whole wheat flour, sugar, all-purpose flour, poppy seeds, baking powder, baking soda, and salt in a large bowl and whisk to mix well.

3. Combine the buttermilk, remaining 1/4 cup oil, the egg, vanilla, and orange zest in a medium bowl and whisk until smooth. Add the buttermilk mixture to the flour mixture, stirring just until moistened. Spread half of the batter into the prepared pan. Top with the blueberries. Dollop the remaining batter over the blueberries, leaving some of the berries uncovered. Bake until the top is lightly browned, 35 to 40 minutes.

4. Cool the cake in the pan on a wire rack for 10 minutes. Run a thin-bladed knife around the edge of the case and remove from the pan. Serve the cake warm or at room temperature. The cake is best on the day it is made.

Nutrition Info:

27 g carb, 174 cal, 6 g fat, 1 g sat fat, 19 mg chol, 2 g fib, 3 g pro, 109 mg sod •
Carb Choices: 2; Exchanges: 2 carb, 1 fat

Pear And Walnut Stuffing

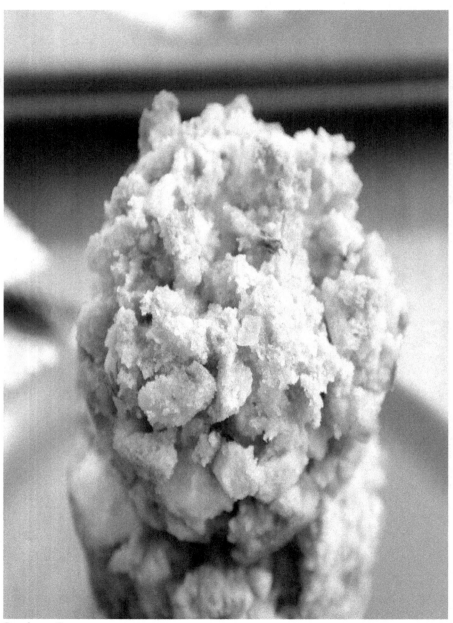

Servings: 8

Ingredients:

6 cups 1/2-inch whole grain bread cubes

3 teaspoons extra virgin olive oil, divided

1 small onion, diced

1 carrot, peeled and diced 1 stalk celery, diced

2 large ripe pears (about 1 pound), peeled, cored, and chopped

2 teaspoons chopped fresh thyme or 1/2 teaspoon dried thyme

1/4 teaspoon kosher salt

1/8 teaspoon freshly ground pepper

1/3 cup walnuts, toasted and chopped

1 1/2 cups Chicken Stock or low-sodium chicken broth

Directions:

1. Preheat the oven to 350°F. Place the bread cubes in a single layer on a large rimmed baking sheet. Bake, stirring once, until the cubes are lightly toasted, 12 to 15 minutes. Set aside. Maintain the oven temperature.

2. Brush a 2-quart baking dish with 1 teaspoon of the oil.

3. Heat a large nonstick skillet over medium heat. Add the remaining 2 teaspoons oil and tilt the pan to coat the bottom evenly. Add the onion, carrot, and celery and cook, stirring often, until the vegetables are softened, 8 minutes. Stir in the pears and cook, stirring occasionally, until they begin to soften, 5 minutes. Stir in the thyme, salt, and pepper. Transfer the vegetable mixture to a large bowl and stir in the bread cubes and walnuts. Add the stock and stir until the stock is absorbed.

4. Spoon the stuffing into the prepared baking dish, cover with foil, and bake 20 minutes. Uncover and bake until the top of the stuffing is lightly browned, about 15 minutes longer. Serve at once.

Nutrition Info:

22 g carb, 153 cal, 6 g fat, 1 g sat fat, 1 mg chol, 8 g fib, 4 g pro, 157 mg sod • Carb Choices: 1 1/2; Exchanges: 1 starch, 1/2 fruit, 1 fat

Fresh Fruit Trifle

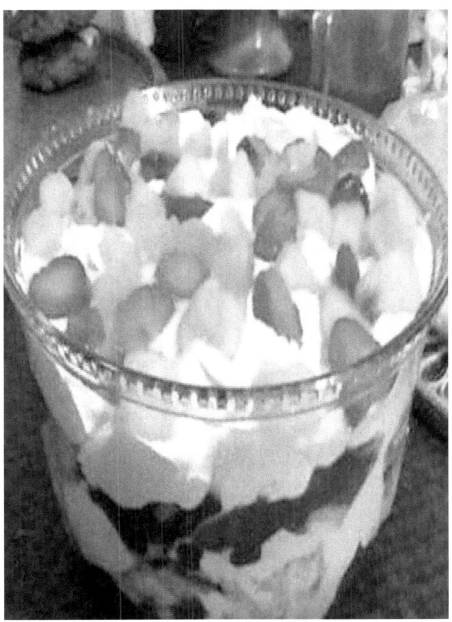

Servings: 16

Ingredients:

2 large oranges

1 Moist Yogurt Cake, prepared, cooled, and cut into 1-inch cubes

2 recipes Vanilla Pudding, prepared and cooled to room temperature

2 cups sliced fresh strawberries

1 medium banana, sliced

2 tablespoons flaked sweetened coconut

Directions:

1. Cut a thin slice from the top and bottom of the oranges, exposing the flesh. Stand each orange upright, and using a sharp knife, thickly cut off the peel, following the contour of the fruit and removing all the white pith and membrane. Holding each orange over a bowl, carefully cut along both sides of each section to free it from the membrane. Discard any seeds and let the sections fall into the bowl.

2. To assemble the trifle, arrange one-third of the cake cubes in a 4-quart trifle bowl, top with one-third of the pudding, one-third of the oranges, one- third of the strawberries, and one-third of the banana slices. Repeat the layering twice with the remaining ingredients. Sprinkle the trifle with the coconut. Serve the trifle at room temperature or chilled. The trifle tastes best on the day it is made.

Nutrition Info:

35 g carb, 202 cal, 5 g fat, 3 g sat fat, 51 mg chol, 1 g fib, 5 g pro, 167 mg sod •
Carb Choices: 2; Exchanges: 2 carb, 1/2 fruit, 1 fat

Smoky Red Pepper–orange Sauce

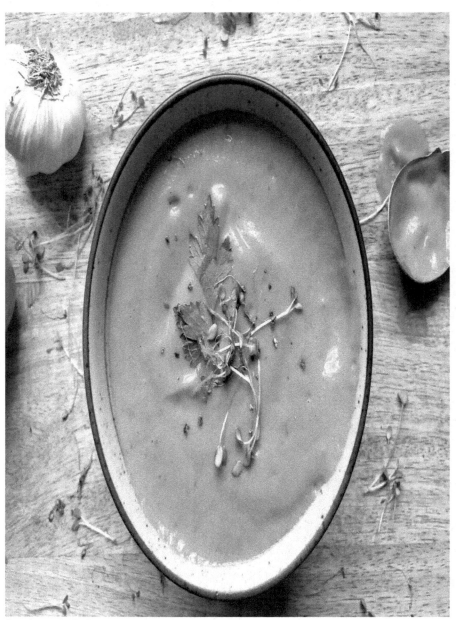

Servings: 11/4 Cups

Ingredients:

1 large red Roasted Bell Pepper or 1 cup roasted red peppers from a jar, chopped

1/3 cup frozen orange juice concentrate, thawed

1 tablespoon extra virgin olive oil

1 tablespoon lime juice

1/2 teaspoon minced chipotle in adobo sauce

1/2 teaspoon ground cumin

1/4 teaspoon kosher salt

Directions:

1. Combine all the ingredients in a food processor and process until smooth. Serve at once, or cover and refrigerate for up to 4 days.

Nutrition Info:

5 g carb, 34 cal, 2 g fat, 0 g sat fat, 0 mg chol, 0 g fib, 0 g pro, 47 mg sod • Carb Choices: 0

Beer-braised Beef Brisket

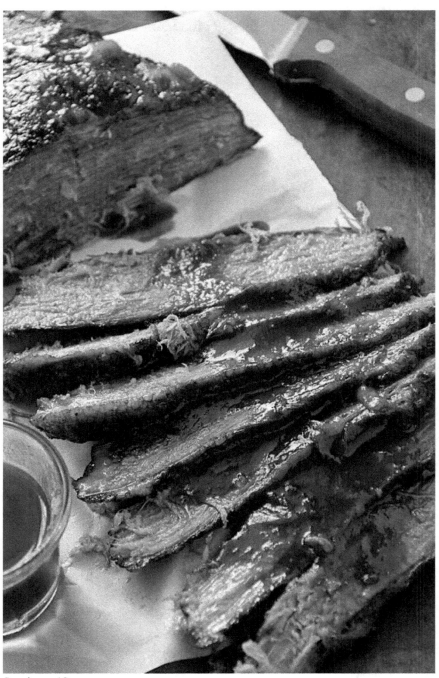

Servings: 12

Ingredients:

1 (3-pound) flat half beef brisket, trimmed of all visible fat

1 teaspoon kosher salt, divided

1/4 teaspoon freshly ground pepper

4 teaspoons extra virgin olive oil, divided

2 large onions, thinly sliced

2 garlic cloves, minced

1 (12-ounce) bottle dark beer, at room temperature

2 tablespoons no-salt-added tomato paste

1 bay leaf

1 teaspoon balsamic vinegar

Directions:

1. Preheat the oven to 325°F.

2. Sprinkle the brisket with 3⁄4 teaspoon of the salt and the pepper. Heat a large Dutch oven over medium-high heat. Add 2 teaspoons of the oil and the brisket and cook, turning to brown on both sides, 6 to 8 minutes. Transfer the brisket to a plate.

3. Add the remaining 2 teaspoons oil to the Dutch oven and tilt the pan to coat the bottom evenly. Add the onions and cook, stirring often, until lightly browned, 8 to 10 minutes. Add the garlic and cook, stirring constantly, until fragrant, 30 seconds. Add the beer, tomato paste, bay leaf and remaining 1⁄4 teaspoon salt and cook, stirring to scrape up the browned bits from the bottom of the pot.

4. Return the brisket to the pot. Cover and bake until the roast is very tender, 21⁄2 to 3 hours. Transfer the roast to a cutting board. Stir the vinegar into the onion mixture in the Dutch oven. Remove and discard the bay leaf. Slice the roast across the grain into thick slices and divide evenly among 12 plates. Spoon the onion mixture evenly over the roast and serve at once.

Nutrition Info:

4 g carb, 184 cal, 6 g fat, 2 g sat fat, 48 mg chol, 1 g fib, 24 g pro, 136 mg sod • Carb Choices: 0; Exchanges: 3 lean protein

Artichoke, Feta, And Olive Pizza

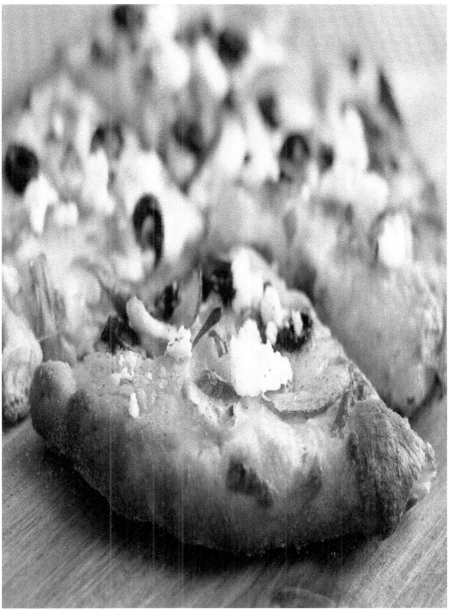

Servings: 4

Ingredients:

1 cup canned artichoke hearts, drained

1 prepared Whole Wheat Pizza Crust or 1 (12-inch) purchased pre-baked whole wheat thin pizza crust

1 recipe Roasted Red Pepper Pizza Sauce

2 tablespoons thinly sliced pitted Kalamata olives

2 ounces finely crumbled feta cheese (about 1/2 cup)

Directions:

1. Position an oven rack on the lowest rung of the oven. Preheat the oven to 450°F.

2. Cut the artichokes into quarters. Place on several thicknesses of paper towels and gently blot dry. Set aside.

3. Place the crust on the bottom rack of the oven and bake 5 minutes.

4. Remove the crust from the oven and spread the sauce evenly over the crust, leaving a 1/2-inch border. Arrange the artichokes evenly over the sauce. Sprinkle with the olives, then with the feta. Bake on the bottom rack until the crust is browned and the cheese melts, about 8 minutes. Cut into 8 wedges and serve at once.

Nutrition Info:

37 g carb, 248 cal, 9 g fat, 3 g sat fat, 13 mg chol, 5 g fib, 9 g pro, 579 mg sod •
Carb Choices: 21/2; Exchanges: 2 starch, 1 veg, 11/2 fat

Pizza with Fresh Tomatoes And Mozzarella

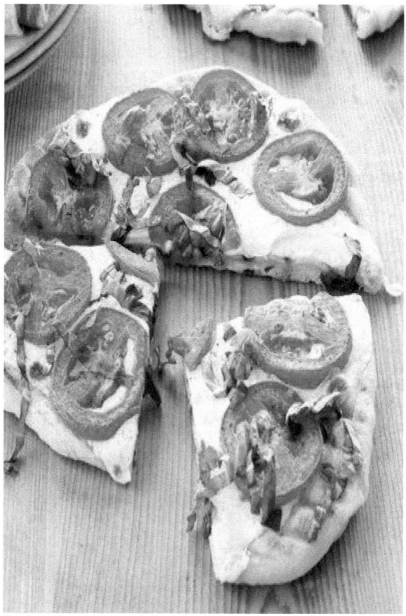

Servings: 4

Ingredients:

1 prepared Whole Wheat Pizza Crust or 1 (12-inch) purchased prebaked whole wheat thin pizza crust

1 recipe Pizza Sauce

2 plum tomatoes, thinly sliced

3 ounces fresh mozzarella, cut into small cubes, or 3/4 cup shredded part- skim mozzarella

4 basil leaves, thinly sliced

Directions:

1. Position an oven rack on the lowest rung of the oven. Preheat the oven to 450°F.
2. Place the crust on the bottom rack of the oven and bake 5 minutes. Remove the crust from the oven and spread the sauce evenly over the crust, leaving a 1/2-inch border. Arrange the tomato slices evenly over the sauce in a single layer. Sprinkle with the mozzarella. Bake on the bottom rack until the crust is browned and the cheese melts, about 8 minutes. Sprinkle with the basil, cut into 8 wedges, and serve at once.

Nutrition Info:

37 g carb, 273 cal, 11 g fat, 2 g sat fat, 8 mg chol, 5 g fib, 11 g pro, 205 mg sod • Carb Choices: 21/2; Exchanges: 2 starch, 1 veg, 2 fat

Cucumber-mango Salad

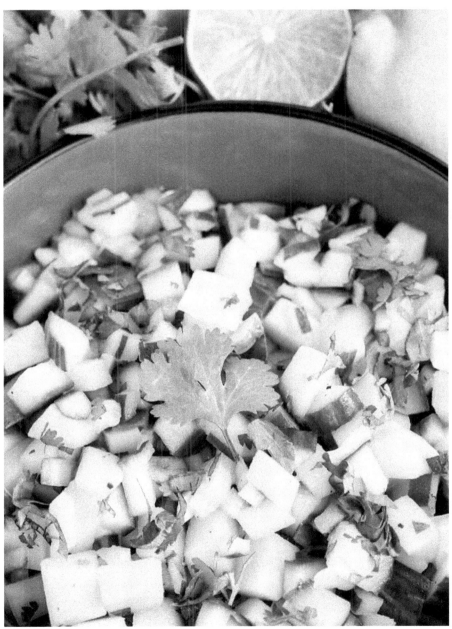

Servings: 4

Ingredients:

1 teaspoon grated lime zest

2 tablespoons lime juice

1 tablespoon canola oil

1 teaspoon honey

1/2 teaspoon kosher salt

1/4 teaspoon ground cumin

1/4 teaspoon ground coriander

Pinch of ground cayenne

1 large mango, peeled, pitted, and thinly sliced

1 hothouse (English) cucumber, halved lengthwise, seeded, and cut into thin strips

1 medium red bell pepper, thinly sliced

1/4 cup chopped fresh cilantro

Directions:

1. Whisk together the lime zest, lime juice, oil, honey, salt, cumin, coriander, and cayenne in a large bowl.

2. Add the mango, cucumber, bell pepper, and cilantro and toss to coat. Serve at once, or cover, and refrigerate up to 1 day. Let stand at room temperature 30 minutes before serving.

Nutrition Info:

14 g carb, 88 cal, 4 g fat, 0 g sat fat, 0 mg chol, 2 g fib, 1 g pro, 143 mg sod • Carb Choices: 1; Exchanges: 1/2 fruit, 1 veg, 1/2 fat

Shiitake Mushrooms with Ginger

Servings: 4

Ingredients:

1 1/2 pounds shiitake mushrooms

3 tablespoons Chicken Stock or low-sodium chicken broth

2 tablespoons reduced-sodium soy sauce

1 1/2 teaspoons rice vinegar

1/2 teaspoon cornstarch

1/2 teaspoon sugar

1/2 teaspoon chili-garlic paste

1/4 teaspoon kosher salt

2 teaspoons canola oil

1 tablespoon minced fresh ginger

1 scallion, thinly sliced

Directions:

1. Remove and discard the tough stems from the mushrooms and slice the caps.

2. Stir together the stock, soy sauce, vinegar, cornstarch, sugar, chili-garlic paste, and salt in a small bowl and set aside.

3. Heat a large wok or nonstick skillet over medium-high heat. Add the oil and tilt the pan to coat the bottom evenly. Add the ginger and cook, stirring constantly, until fragrant, 30 seconds.

4. Add the mushrooms and cook, stirring constantly, until softened, about 5 minutes. Stir the stock mixture and add to the skillet. Cook, stirring constantly, until the sauce comes to a boil and thickens slightly, 1 minute. Stir in the scallion. Spoon the mushrooms into a serving dish and serve at once.

Nutrition Info:

15 g carb, 82 cal, 3 g fat, 0 g sat fat, 0 mg chol, 2 g fib, 2 g pro, 409 mg sod • Carb Choices: 1; Exchanges: 3 veg, 1/2 fat

Pasta, Turkey Sausage, And White Beans In Garlicky Tomato Sauce C

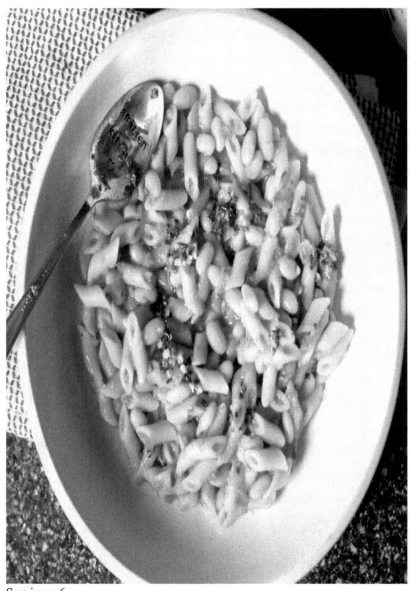

Servings: 6

Ingredients:

4 ounces whole wheat penne or other short pasta (about 1 1/2 cups)

4 teaspoons extra virgin olive oil, divided

8 ounces Italian turkey sausage, cut into 1 1/2-inch slices

1 medium onion, chopped

4 garlic cloves, minced

1 (28-ounce) can no-salt-added whole tomatoes, undrained and chopped

1 (15-ounce) can no-salt-added cannellini beans, rinsed and drained

1/8 teaspoon freshly ground pepper

2 tablespoons chopped fresh Italian parsley

3 tablespoons freshly grated Parmesan

Directions:

1. Cook the pasta according to the package directions.

2. Meanwhile, heat a large nonstick skillet over medium heat. Add 2 teaspoons of the oil and tilt the pan to coat the bottom evenly. Add the sausage and cook, turning often, until well browned, about 6 minutes. Transfer to a plate.

3. Add the remaining 2 teaspoons oil and tilt the pan to coat the bottom evenly. Add the onion and cook, stirring occasionally, until softened, 5 minutes. Add the garlic and cook, stirring constantly, until fragrant, 30 seconds.

4. Stir in the tomatoes and their juices, the beans, pepper, and the sausage and bring to a boil. Reduce the heat to low, cover, and simmer 15 minutes. Add the pasta and parsley and stir to combine. Spoon the pasta mixture evenly onto 6 plates, sprinkle evenly with the Parmesan, and serve at once.

Nutrition Info:

32 g carb, 242 cal, 8 g fat, 1 g sat fat, 19 mg chol, 6 g fib, 13 g pro, 264 mg sod • Carb Choices: 2; Exchanges: 1 1/2 starch, 1 veg, 1 medium-fat protein, 1 lean protein, 1/2 fat

Barley Risotto with Spinach And Feta

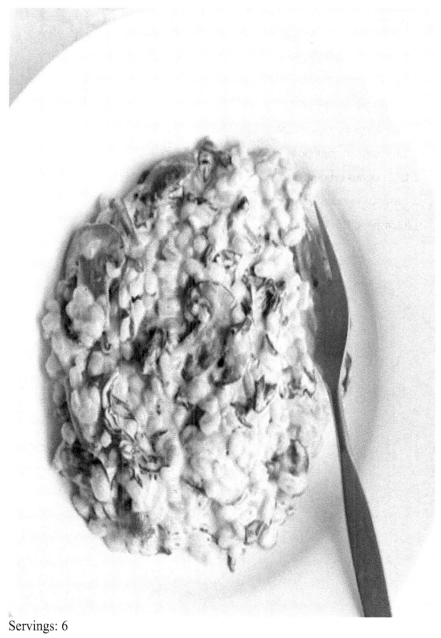

Servings: 6

Ingredients:

4 1/2 cups Vegetable Stock or low-sodium vegetable broth

2 teaspoons extra virgin olive oil

1/2 cup minced shallots

3/4 cup pearl barley

1/2 cup dry white wine

1/2 teaspoon kosher salt

2 cups chopped fresh spinach

1 large tomato, chopped

2 tablespoons crumbled feta cheese

2 teaspoons grated lemon zest

1/8 teaspoon freshly ground pepper

Directions:

1. Pour the stock into a medium saucepan and bring to a simmer over medium-high heat. Reduce the heat to low and keep the stock warm.

2. Heat a large saucepan over medium heat. Add the oil and tilt the pan to coat the bottom evenly. Add the shallots and cook, stirring often, until softened, 5 minutes.

3. Add the barley and cook, stirring constantly, 2 minutes. Add the wine and salt and cook, stirring frequently until absorbed. Add the stock, 1/2 cup at a time, stirring frequently, until the liquid is absorbed after each addition before adding more. When all the liquid is absorbed and the barley is tender, yet firm to the bite (about 35 minutes), add the spinach, tomato, and feta and cook, stirring constantly, until the spinach is wilted and the tomato is heated through, about 2 minutes. Remove from the heat and stir in the lemon zest and pepper. Spoon the risotto into a serving dish and serve at once.

Nutrition Info:

26 g carb, 159 cal, 3 g fat, 1 g sat fat, 3 mg chol, 5 g fib, 4 g pro, 247 mg sod • Carb Choices: 2; Exchanges: 2 starch, 1/2 fat

Ricotta Pancakes with Fresh Strawberries

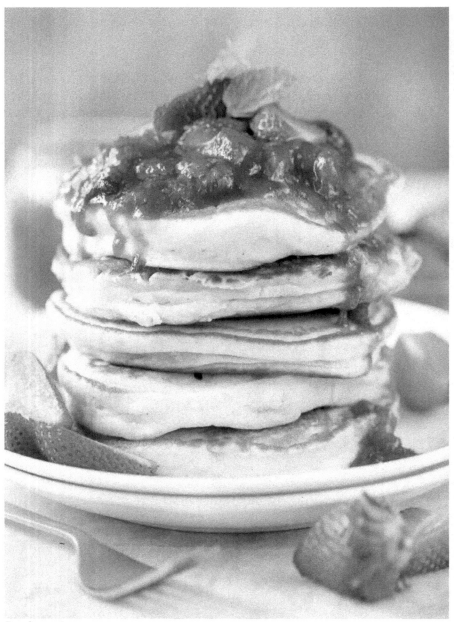

Servings: 6

Ingredients:

1 cup part-skim ricotta

1/3 cup skim milk

2 large eggs, separated

1/3 cup unbleached all-purpose flour

1 tablespoon granulated sugar

2 teaspoons grated orange zest

Pinch of salt

1 1/2 teaspoons canola oil, divided

2 teaspoons confectioners' sugar

3 cups sliced fresh strawberries

Directions:

1. Preheat the oven to 250°F. Place a large baking sheet in the oven.

2. Combine the ricotta, milk, egg yolks, flour, granulated sugar, orange zest, and salt in a large bowl and whisk until smooth.

3. Place the egg whites in a large bowl and beat at high speed with an electric mixer until stiff peaks form. Fold the egg whites into the ricotta mixture in 3 additions, stirring until no white streaks appear.

4. Heat a large nonstick griddle or large nonstick skillet over medium heat. Brush with 1/2 teaspoon of the oil using a silicone brush. Spoon the batter by scant 1/4-cup measures onto the griddle 4 at a time. Turn the pancakes when the tops are covered with bubbles and the edges look cooked. Place the pancakes on the baking sheet in the oven to keep warm. Repeat the procedure with the remaining oil and batter to make 12 pancakes.

5. Place 2 pancakes on each plate. Sprinkle the pancakes evenly with the confectioners' sugar. Accompany each serving with 1/2 cup of the strawberries.

Nutrition Info:

17 g carb, 156 cal, 6 g fat, 3 g sat fat, 84 mg chol, 2 g fib, 8 g pro, 106 mg sod • Carb Choices: 1; Exchanges: 1 starch, 1 fat

Icy Cold Melon-mint Soup

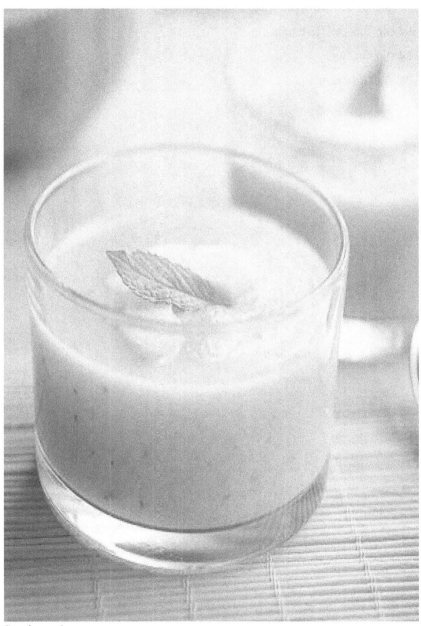

Servings: 6

Ingredients:

1 large cantaloupe, seeded, peeled, and chopped (about 8 cups)

1 cup unsweetened apple juice

1/4 cup chopped fresh mint

1/4 cup lime juice

Pinch of kosher salt

Directions:

1. Combine all the ingredients in a food processor or blender and process until smooth. Cover and refrigerate until chilled, 2 hours or up to 8 hours. Ladle into 6 bowls and serve.

Nutrition Info:

23 g carb, 95 cal, 0 g fat, 0 g sat fat, 0 mg chol, 2 g fib, 2 g pro, 48 mg sod • Carb Choices: 1 1/2; Exchanges: 1 1/2 fruit

Thai Rice Noodle Salad

Servings: 6

Ingredients:

6 ounces thin rice noodles

3 tablespoons lime juice

2 tablespoons Asian fish sauce

1 tablespoon canola oil

1/2 teaspoon sugar

1/4 teaspoon chili-garlic paste

1 carrot, peeled and coarsely shredded

1 shallot, thinly sliced or 1/4 cup thinly sliced red onion

1/2 medium hothouse (English) cucumber, diced

2 tablespoons chopped fresh mint

2 tablespoons chopped fresh cilantro

3 tablespoons dry-roasted peanuts, chopped

Directions:

1. Cook the noodles according to the package directions. Drain in a colander and rinse under cold running water until cool. Drain well.

2. Meanwhile, whisk together the lime juice, fish sauce, oil, sugar, and chili-garlic paste in a large bowl. Add the cooked noodles, carrot, shallot, cucumber, mint, and cilantro and toss to coat. Refrigerate the salad, covered, until chilled, 2 hours or up to 1 day. Sprinkle with the peanuts just before serving.

Nutrition Info:

31 g carb, 177 cal, 5 g fat, 1 g sat fat, 0 mg chol, 1 g fib, 4 g pro, 482 mg sod • Carb Choices: 2; Exchanges: 1 1/2 starch, 1 veg, 1 fat

White Bean Salad with Tomatoes And Sage

Servings: 4

Ingredients:

2 tablespoon extra virgin olive oil

1 garlic clove, minced

1 tablespoon minced fresh sage or 1 teaspoon crumbled dried sage

2 tablespoons red wine vinegar

1 teaspoon Dijon mustard

1/2 teaspoon kosher salt

1/8 teaspoon freshly ground pepper

1 (15-ounce) can no-salt-added cannellini beans, rinsed and drained

2 plum tomatoes, each cut into 8 wedges

Directions:

1. Combine the oil, garlic, and sage in a small saucepan. Set over medium- low heat and cook, stirring often, until the oil is warmed and the garlic and sage are fragrant, about 3 minutes. Transfer to a large bowl to cool.

2. Whisk the vinegar, mustard, salt, and pepper into the oil mixture. Add the beans and tomatoes and toss gently to combine. Serve the salad at room temperature. The salad tastes best on the day it is made, but it can be refrigerated, covered, for up to 1 day. Let stand at room temperature 30 minutes before serving.

Nutrition Info:

17 g carb, 160 cal, 8 g fat, 1 g sat fat, 0 mg chol, 5 g fib, 6 g pro, 207 mg sod • Carb Choices: 1; Exchanges: 1 starch, 1 plant-based protein, 1 1/2 fat

Lemongrass-ginger Baked Chicken

Servings: 4

Ingredients:

1 teaspoon canola oil

1 cup cilantro leaves

1/4 cup chopped fresh ginger

3 tablespoons thinly sliced lemongrass

2 tablespoons reduced-sodium soy sauce

2 garlic cloves, chopped

1 jalapeño, seeded and chopped

4 (6-ounce) bone-in skin-on chicken breasts

Lime wedges

Directions:

1. Preheat the oven to 375°F. Brush a medium roasting pan with the oil.

2. Combine the cilantro, ginger, lemongrass, soy sauce, garlic, and jalapeño in a food processor and process until the mixture forms a finely minced paste (add a tablespoon or two of water, if necessary, to achieve the desired consistency).

3. Gently loosen but do not detach the skin from the chicken breasts. Rub the cilantro paste over the breast underneath the skin. Arrange the chicken skin side up in the prepared pan. Bake until the juices of the chicken run clear, 30 to 35 minutes. Divide the chicken among 4 plates and serve at once with the lime wedges. Remove the skin before eating.

Nutrition Info:

3 g carb, 159 cal, 4 g fat, 1 g sat fat, 68 mg chol, 0 g fib, 26 g pro, 365 mg sod • Carb Choices: 0; Exchanges: 4 lean protein

Huevos Rancheros

Servings: 4

Ingredients:

2 teaspoons canola oil

1 poblano chile, seeded and chopped

1 small onion, chopped

2 garlic cloves, minced

1/2 teaspoon ground cumin

1 (14-ounce) can no-salt-added whole tomatoes, undrained and chopped

1/4 teaspoon kosher salt

1/8 teaspoon freshly ground pepper

2 tablespoons chopped fresh cilantro

4 large eggs

1 tablespoon white vinegar

4 (6-inch) whole wheat flour tortillas, warmed

1 ounce shredded reduced-fat sharp Cheddar cheese (about 1/4 cup)

Directions:

1. Heat a large nonstick skillet over medium heat. Add the oil and tilt the pan to coat the bottom evenly. Add the chile and onion, and cook, stirring often, until softened, 5 minutes. Add the garlic and cumin and cook, stirring constantly, until fragrant, 30 seconds.

2. Stir in the tomatoes and their juices, the salt, and pepper and bring to a boil over high heat. Reduce the heat to low, cover, and simmer 10 minutes. Uncover and simmer until the sauce is slightly thickened, 5 minutes longer. Stir in the cilantro.

3. When the sauce is almost done, prepare the eggs. Fill a large deep skillet or broad saucepan with 3 inches of water. Add the vinegar and bring to a boil. Reduce the heat until the water is just at a simmer and break the eggs into the water. Turn off the heat, cover, and let stand 2 to 3 minutes.

4. Place 1 tortilla on each plate. Using a slotted spoon, top each tortilla with a poached egg. Spoon the sauce evenly over the eggs and sprinkle evenly with the Cheddar. Serve at once.

Nutrition Info:

20 g carb, 225 cal, 11 g fat, 3 g sat fat, 217 mg chol, 10 g fib, 12 g pro, 395 mg sod
• Carb Choices: 1; Exchanges: 1/2 starch, 1 veg, 1 medium-fat protein, 1/2 fat

Eye Of Round with Roasted Garlic–horseradish Sauce

Servings: 8

Ingredients:

1/2 cup dry red wine

1/4 cup red wine vinegar

1 small onion, thinly sliced

4 garlic cloves, minced

2 teaspoons whole black peppercorns, crushed

1 (2-pound) eye of round roast, trimmed of all visible fat

1 head garlic

1 1/4 teaspoons kosher salt, divided

2 teaspoons extra virgin olive oil

1/2 cup plain low-fat Greek yogurt or strained yogurt

2 tablespoons mayonnaise

1 tablespoon prepared horseradish, drained

1 teaspoon lemon juice

Directions:

1. To make the roast, combine the wine, vinegar, onion, minced garlic, and peppercorns in a large resealable plastic bag. Add the roast, seal the bag, and refrigerate 8 hours and up to 24 hours.
2. Preheat the oven to 325°F.
3. Separate the head of garlic into cloves, but do not peel. Place on a sheet of foil and wrap tightly. Place in a small baking dish.
4. Remove the roast from the marinade and discard the marinade. Pat the roast dry with paper towels. Sprinkle the roast with 1 teaspoon of the salt.
5. Heat a large heavy-bottomed ovenproof skillet over medium-high heat. Add the oil and tilt the pan to coat the bottom evenly. Cook the roast, turning occasionally, until well browned on all sides, about 6 minutes.
6. Place the roast and the prepared head of garlic in the oven. Bake the roast, turning once, until an instant-read thermometer inserted into the center reads 145°F, and the garlic is very soft, 40 to 45 minutes. Cover the roast loosely with foil and let stand about 10 minutes.
7. Meanwhile, to make the sauce, unwrap the garlic and let stand until cool enough to handle. Squeeze the garlic pulp from each clove into a small bowl. Whisk in the yogurt, mayonnaise, horseradish, lemon juice, and the remaining 1/4 teaspoon salt. Cut the beef into thin slices and divide evenly among 8 plates. Serve with the sauce.

Nutrition Info:

3 g carb, 197 cal, 8 g fat, 2 g sat fat, 50 mg chol, 0 g fib, 26 g pro, 278 mg sod •
Carb Choices: 0; Exchanges: 3 lean protein, 1/2 fat

Tex-mex Cheddar, Polenta, And Vegetable Casserole

Servings: 6

Ingredients:

3 teaspoons canola oil, divided

1 medium onion, diced

1 medium red bell pepper, diced

1 medium zucchini, diced

1 jalapeño, seeded and minced

2 cloves garlic, minced

2 teaspoons chili powder

1 teaspoon ground cumin

2 cups Vegetable Stock or low-sodium vegetable broth

1/2 teaspoon kosher salt

1/2 cup fine-grind yellow cornmeal

3 large egg whites

4 ounces shredded reduced-fat sharp Cheddar cheese (about 1 cup)

2 large eggs

1/4 cup chopped fresh cilantro

Directions:

1. Preheat the oven to 375°F. Brush an 11 x 7-inch baking dish with 1 teaspoon of the oil.
2. Heat a large nonstick skillet over medium-high heat. Add the remaining 2 teaspoons oil and tilt the pan to coat. Add the onion, bell pepper, zucchini, and jalapeño and cook, stirring occasionally, until the vegetables are tender, 8 to 10 minutes. Add the garlic, chili powder, and cumin and cook, stirring constantly, until fragrant, 1 minute longer. Transfer the vegetable mixture to a bowl. Do not wash the skillet.
3. Add the broth and salt to the skillet and bring to a boil. Slowly whisk in the cornmeal and cook, whisking constantly, until the polenta is thickened, 2 to 3 minutes. Transfer the polenta to a large bowl and let stand to cool slightly.
4. Place the egg whites in a large bowl and beat at high speed with an electric mixer until stiff peaks form. Stir the vegetable mixture, Cheddar, eggs, and cilantro into the polenta. Fold the egg whites into the polenta mixture in 3 additions, stirring until no white streaks appear.
5. Spoon into the prepared baking dish and bake for 30 minutes or until the center is set and the edges are lightly browned. Let stand 5 minutes before serving. Spoon the casserole evenly onto 6 plates and serve at once.

Nutrition Info:

16 g carb, 181 cal, 8 g fat, 3 g sat fat, 84 mg chol, 2 g fib, 10 g pro, 357 mg sod •
Carb Choices: 1; Exchanges: 1/2 starch, 1 veg, 1 high-fat protein, 1/2 fat

Nicoise Pasta Salad

Servings: 6

Ingredients:

6 ounces whole wheat penne or other short pasta (about 2 cups)

8 ounces green beans, trimmed and cut into 2-inch pieces

2 (5-ounce) cans low-sodium chunk white albacore tuna in water, drained and flaked

1 1/2 cups cherry or grape tomatoes, halved

1/4 cup nicoise or other oil-cured black olives, pitted and halved

1/4 cup chopped fresh Italian parsley

3 tablespoons minced red onion

3 tablespoons capers, rinsed and drained

1 recipe Basic Vinaigrette

Directions:

1. Cook the pasta according to the package directions, adding the green beans during the last 4 minutes of cooking. Drain in a colander and rinse with cold running water until cool.

2. Combine the pasta and beans, tuna, tomatoes, olives, parsley, onion, and capers in a large bowl. Drizzle with the vinaigrette and toss to coat. Serve the salad at room temperature. The salad tastes best on the day it is made, but it can be refrigerated, covered, for up to 1 day. Let stand at room temperature 30 minutes before serving.

Nutrition Info:

26 g carb, 208 cal, 7 g fat, 1 g sat fat, 17 mg chol, 4 g fib, 16 g pro, 273 mg sod • Carb Choices: 2; Exchanges: 1 1/2 starch, 1 veg, 1 lean protein, 1 1/2 fat

Fish Fillets with Quick Tomato-dill Sauce

Servings: 4

Ingredients:

1/4 cup unbleached all-purpose flour

4 (5-ounce) thin white-fleshed fish fillets

1/4 teaspoon plus pinch of kosher salt, divided

1/8 teaspoon plus pinch of freshly ground pepper, divided

4 teaspoons extra virgin olive oil, divided

1/4 cup diced onion

1 large tomato, chopped

1 tablespoon chopped fresh dill

1 teaspoon grated lemon zest

Directions:

1. Place the flour on a plate. Sprinkle the fish fillets with 1/4 teaspoon of the salt and 1/8 teaspoon of the pepper, then dip each one in the flour.

2. Heat a large nonstick skillet over medium heat. Add 2 teaspoons of the oil and tilt the pan to coat the bottom evenly. Add the fish and cook, turning once, until the fish flakes when tested with a fork, about 3 minutes on each side. Transfer to a plate and cover loosely with foil to keep warm.

3. Add the remaining 2 teaspoons oil and tilt the pan to coat the bottom evenly. Add the onion, and cook, stirring often, just until softened, about 3 minutes. Add the tomato and cook, stirring often, until heated through, about 2 minutes. Remove from the heat and stir in the dill, lemon zest, and the remaining pinch of salt and pinch of pepper. Divide the fish among 4 plates, spoon the sauce evenly over the fish, and serve at once.

Nutrition Info:

7 g carb, 191 cal, 6 g fat, 1 g sat fat, 67 mg chol, 1 g fib, 25 g pro, 193 mg sod • Carb Choices: 1/2; Exchanges: 1/2 carb, 3 lean protein, 1 fat

White Bean, Artichoke, And Zucchini Stew

Servings: 6

Ingredients:

2 teaspoons extra virgin olive oil

1 medium onion, chopped

1 medium red bell pepper, chopped

2 garlic cloves, chopped

3 cups Vegetable Stock or low-sodium vegetable broth

2 (15-ounce) cans no-salt-added cannellini beans, rinsed and drained

1 (141/2-ounce) can no-salt-added diced tomatoes, drained

1/4 cup no-salt-added tomato paste

2 teaspoons chopped fresh rosemary

1 (14-ounce) can artichoke hearts

1 medium zucchini, quartered lengthwise and sliced

2 cups chopped fresh spinach

11/2 teaspoons balsamic vinegar

Pinch of crushed red pepper

Directions:

1. Heat a large pot over medium heat. Add the oil and tilt the pan to coat the bottom evenly. Add the onion and bell pepper and cook, stirring often, until the vegetables are softened, 5 minutes. Add the garlic and cook, stirring constantly, until fragrant, 30 seconds. Add the stock, beans, tomatoes, tomato paste, and rosemary and bring to a boil over high heat. Cover, reduce the heat, and simmer until the vegetables are tender, 15 minutes.

2. Meanwhile, drain and rinse the artichoke hearts and cut into quarters. Place the artichokes on several thicknesses of paper towels and gently blot dry.

3. Add the artichoke hearts and zucchini to the pot and return to a simmer. Cook until the zucchini is crisp-tender, about 3 minutes. Stir in the spinach and cook just until the spinach wilts, about 1 minute. Stir in the vinegar and crushed red pepper. Ladle the stew evenly into 6 bowls and serve at once.

Nutrition Info:

34 g carb, 201 cal, 3 g fat, 0 g sat fat, 0 mg chol, 8 g fib, 10 g pro, 311 mg sod • Carb Choices: 2; Exchanges: 1 starch, 3 veg, 1 plant-based protein

Parmesan-rosemary Wheat Loaf

Servings: 16

Ingredients:

1 cup lukewarm water

1 package active dry yeast

21/4 to 21/2 cups whole wheat flour

2 ounces freshly grated Parmesan (about 1/2 cup)

2 tablespoons plus 1 teaspoon canola oil, divided

1 tablespoon sugar

1 tablespoon chopped fresh rosemary

1 teaspoon salt

1/8 teaspoon freshly ground pepper

Directions:

1. Combine the water and yeast in a large bowl and stir until the yeast dissolves. Let stand 5 minutes. Add 2 1/4 cups of the flour, the Parmesan, 2 tablespoons of the oil, the sugar, rosemary, salt, and pepper and stir until a soft dough forms.

2. Turn the dough out onto a lightly floured surface. Knead until smooth and elastic, about 8 minutes. Add enough of the remaining 1/4 cup flour, 1 tablespoon at a time, to prevent the dough from sticking to your hands. (Alternatively, knead the dough for 5 minutes at low speed with an electric mixer using a dough hook, adding enough of the remaining 1/4 cup flour, 1 tablespoon at a time, to make a smooth dough.)

3. Brush a large bowl with the remaining 1 teaspoon oil. Place the dough in the bowl and turn to coat the top. Cover and let rise in a warm place (85°F), free from drafts, until doubled in size, about 1 hour.

4. Line a 9 x 5-inch loaf pan with parchment paper. Place the dough in the prepared pan. Cover loosely with lightly oiled plastic wrap and let rise in a warm place (85°F), free from drafts, until doubled in size, about 45 minutes.

5. Preheat the oven to 350°F. Remove the plastic wrap and bake the loaf 20 minutes. Cover loosely with foil and bake until the loaf is golden brown and sounds hollow when tapped, about 10 minutes longer.

6. Cool the bread in the pan on a wire rack for 10 minutes. Remove from the pan and cool completely on a wire rack. Slice using a serrated knife. The bread can be stored inside a paper bag at room temperature for up to 2 days or frozen for up to 3 months.

Nutrition Info:

15 g carb, 101 cal, 3 g fat, 1 g sat fat, 2 mg chol, 2 g fib, 4 g pro, 184 mg sod • Carb Choices: 1; Exchanges: 1 starch, 1/2 fat

Sweet Potato Puree with Cranberries

Servings: 8

Ingredients:

4 medium sweet potatoes (about 2 1/4 pounds), peeled and cut into 1-inch pieces

3/4 cup fresh cranberries

1/3 cup packed light brown sugar

3 tablespoons orange juice

1/2 teaspoon ground cinnamon

1/4 teaspoon kosher salt

Pinch of ground cloves

1/2 teaspoon vanilla extract

Directions:

1. In a saucepan fitted with a steamer basket, bring 1 inch of water to a boil over high heat. Add the potatoes, reduce the heat to low, cover, and steam until tender, about 15 minutes

2. Meanwhile, combine the cranberries, sugar, orange juice, cinnamon, salt, and cloves in a small saucepan. Bring to a boil over high heat, reduce the heat to low, and simmer until the cranberries pop, about 5 minutes. Remove from the heat and stir in the vanilla.

3. Transfer the potatoes to a large bowl. Mash using a potato masher until smooth. Stir in the cranberry mixture. Serve at once.

Nutrition Info:

26 g carb, 110 cal, 0 g fat, 0 g sat fat, 0 mg chol, 3 g fib, 2 g pro, 66 mg sod • Carb Choices: 2; Exchanges: 1 starch, 1 carb

Braised Lamb with Parsnips And Dried Plums

Servings: 8

Ingredients:

1 teaspoon coriander seeds

2 pounds boneless lamb shoulder, trimmed of all visible fat and cut into 1-inch cubes

3/4 teaspoon ground cinnamon

1/2 teaspoon kosher salt

1/4 teaspoon freshly ground pepper

4 teaspoons extra virgin olive oil, divided

1 large onion, chopped

2 garlic cloves, minced

1 tablespoon minced fresh ginger

4 cups Beef Stock or low-sodium beef broth

1/4 cup no-salt-added tomato paste

3 medium carrots, peeled and chopped

3 medium parsnips, peeled and chopped

1 cup pitted dried plums, halved

Directions:

1. Preheat the oven to 325°F.

2. Place the coriander seeds in a small dry skillet over medium heat and toast, shaking the pan often, until fragrant, about 3 minutes. Transfer to a small dish and allow to cool. Place the seeds in a mortar and crush with a pestle. Alternatively, place the seeds in a small resealable plastic bag. Seal the bag, place on a cutting board, and crush using a meat mallet or the back of a large spoon. Combine the lamb, crushed coriander, cinnamon, salt, and pepper in a large bowl and toss to coat.

3. Heat a Dutch oven over medium-high heat. Add 2 teaspoons of the oil and tilt the pot to coat the bottom evenly. Add half of the lamb and cook, turning occasionally, until browned on all sides, about 6 minutes. Transfer the lamb to a plate. Repeat with the remaining lamb.

4. Add the remaining 2 teaspoons oil to the Dutch oven and tilt the pot to coat the bottom evenly. Add the onion and cook, stirring often, until lightly browned, 8 to 10 minutes. Stir in the garlic and ginger and cook, stirring constantly, until fragrant, 30 seconds. Return the lamb to the Dutch oven. Add the stock and tomato paste. Cover and bake 2 hours. Stir in the carrots, parsnips, and dried plums, cover, and bake until the lamb is very tender, 1 hour longer. Spoon the stew evenly into 8 shallow bowls and serve at once. The stew can be frozen for up to 3 months.

Nutrition Info:

30 g carb, 319 cal, 10 g fat, 3 g sat fat, 79 mg chol, 5 g fib, 28 g pro, 382 mg sod • Carb Choices: 2; Exchanges: 1/2 starch, 1 fruit, 1 veg, 3 lean protein, 1/2 fat

Carrot-ginger Soup

Servings: 4

Ingredients:

2 teaspoons extra virgin olive oil

1 small onion, chopped

2 garlic cloves, chopped

1-pound carrots, peeled and cut into 1-inch slices

3 to 3 1/2 cups Vegetable Stock or low-sodium vegetable broth

1 tablespoon grated fresh ginger

1/4 teaspoon kosher salt

2 tablespoons lime juice

Directions:

1. Heat a large pot over medium heat. Add the oil and tilt the pan to coat the bottom evenly. Add the onion and cook, stirring often, until softened, 5 minutes. Add the garlic and cook, stirring constantly, until fragrant, 30 seconds. Add the carrots, 3 cups of the stock, the ginger, and salt and bring to a boil over high heat. Cover, reduce the heat to low, and simmer until the carrots are very tender, 15 to 20 minutes.

2. Place the carrot mixture in a food processor or blender in batches and process until smooth. Return the soup to the pot and reheat over medium heat. Add the remaining 1/2 cup stock a few tablespoons at a time, if needed, to reach the desired consistency. Stir in the lime juice. Ladle the soup into 4 bowls and serve at once. The soup can be refrigerated, covered, for up to 4 days or frozen for up to 3 months.

Nutrition Info:

15 g carb, 81 cal, 3 g fat, 0 g sat fat, 0 mg chol, 3 g fib, 1 g pro, 321 mg sod • Carb Choices: 1; Exchanges: 3 veg

Braised Baby Artichokes

Servings: 4

Ingredients:

1 small lemon

12 baby artichokes

1 tablespoon extra virgin olive oil

1 small onion, halved and thinly sliced

2 garlic cloves, minced

1/2 cup Chicken Stock or low-sodium chicken broth

1/4 teaspoon kosher salt

1 teaspoon lemon juice

1 tablespoon chopped fresh basil or 1 teaspoon chopped fresh rosemary

Directions:

1. Squeeze the juice from the lemon into a large bowl and fill the bowl three-quarters full with cold water.

2. Working with one at a time, snap off the outer petals of each artichoke until you reach leaves that are half green and half yellow. Cut away and discard the top third of each artichoke. Trim away the brown tip of the stem and peel the stem. Cut each artichoke in half, and remove any pink- or purple-tinted leaves inside. As you finish, place each artichoke in the lemon water.

3. Heat a large skillet over medium heat. Add the oil and tilt the pan to coat the bottom evenly. Add the onion and cook, stirring occasionally, until softened, 5 minutes. Stir in the garlic and cook until fragrant, 30 seconds. Drain the artichokes and add to the pan. Add the stock and salt and bring to a boil over high heat. Cover, reduce the heat to low, and simmer until the artichokes are tender, 8 to 10 minutes. Stir in the lemon juice and basil. Spoon the artichokes into a serving dish. Serve hot, warm, or at room temperature.

Nutrition Info:

12 g carb, 104 cal, 4 g fat, 1 g sat fat, 1 mg chol, 5 g fib, 5 g pro, 202 mg sod • Carb Choices: 1; Exchanges: 2 veg, 1 fat

Butternut Squash Soup

Servings: 6

Ingredients:

2 teaspoons extra virgin olive oil

1 medium onion, chopped

2 carrots, peeled and chopped

2 garlic cloves, minced

1 medium butternut squash, peeled, seeded, and chopped (about 5 cups)

3 to 3 1/2 cups Vegetable Stock or low-sodium vegetable broth

1 teaspoon kosher salt

1 tablespoon lemon juice

Directions:

1. Heat a large pot over medium heat. Add the oil and tilt the pan to coat the bottom evenly. Add the onion and carrots and cook, stirring often, until softened, 5 minutes. Add the garlic and cook, stirring constantly, until fragrant, 30 seconds. Add the squash, 3 cups of the stock, and the salt and bring to a boil over high heat. Cover, reduce the heat to low, and simmer until the squash is very tender, 15 to 20 minutes.

2. Place the squash mixture in a food processor or blender in batches and process until smooth. Return the soup to the pot and reheat gently over medium heat. Add the remaining 1/2 cup stock a few tablespoons at a time, if needed, to reach the desired consistency. Stir in the lemon juice. Ladle the soup into 6 bowls and serve at once. The soup can be refrigerated, covered, for up to 4 days or frozen for up to 3 months.

Nutrition Info:

21 g carb, 95 cal, 2 g fat, 0 g sat fat, 0 mg chol, 4 g fib, 2 g pro, 329 mg sod • Carb Choices: 11/2; Exchanges: 1 starch, 1/2 fruit, 1 veg

Spicy Quinoa with Zucchini And Bell Pepper

Servings: 6

Ingredients:

1 1/2 cups Vegetable Stock or low-sodium vegetable broth

1 cup quinoa, rinsed

1/2 teaspoon kosher salt

2 teaspoons extra virgin olive oil

1/2 cup diced red bell pepper

1/4 cup diced onion

1 jalapeño, seeded and minced

1/2 cup diced zucchini

1 garlic clove, minced

1/2 teaspoon ground cumin

Pinch of ground cayenne

2 tablespoons chopped fresh cilantro

2 teaspoons lime juice

Directions:

1. Combine the stock, quinoa, and salt in a medium saucepan and bring to a boil over high heat. Reduce the heat to low, cover, and simmer until the quinoa is tender, 12 to 15 minutes.

2. Heat a medium nonstick skillet over medium heat. Add the oil and tilt the pan to coat the bottom evenly. Add the bell pepper, onion, and jalapeño and cook, stirring often, until softened, 5 minutes. Add the zucchini, garlic, cumin, and cayenne and cook, stirring often, until the zucchini is crisp-tender, 2 minutes.

3. Remove from the heat and stir in the quinoa, cilantro, and lime juice. Spoon the quinoa into a serving dish and serve at once.

Nutrition Info:

22 g carb, 135 cal, 3 g fat, 0 g sat fat, 0 mg chol, 2 g fib, 4 g pro, 137 mg sod • Carb Choices: 1 1/2; Exchanges: 1 1/2 starch, 1/2 fat

Bean And Cornbread Salad

Servings: 8

Ingredients:

4 cups 1/2-inch cubes Southern Cornbread or purchased cornbread

2 large ears corn, kernels cut from the cob, or 3/4 cup frozen corn kernels

2 tablespoons extra virgin olive oil

1 tablespoon apple cider vinegar

1 teaspoon Dijon mustard

1/2 teaspoon kosher salt

1/4 teaspoon freshly ground pepper

4 scallions, thinly sliced

2 cups cherry tomatoes, quartered

1 (15-ounce) can no-salt-added pinto beans, rinsed and drained

4 ounces shredded reduced-fat sharp Cheddar cheese (about 1 cup)

1 large green or red bell pepper, cut into 1-inch strips

1/2 cup chopped fresh Italian parsley

Directions:

1. Preheat the oven to 350°F. Place the bread cubes in a single layer on a large rimmed baking sheet. Bake, stirring once, until the cubes are lightly toasted, 20 to 25 minutes. Set aside to cool.

2. Meanwhile, fill a medium saucepan half full with water and bring to a boil over high heat. Add the corn and cook 2 minutes. Drain and transfer to a plate to cool.

3. Whisk together the oil, vinegar, mustard, salt, and ground pepper in a large bowl. Add the toasted bread cubes, cooked corn, scallions, tomatoes, beans, Cheddar, bell pepper, and parsley and toss to coat. Serve at once.

Nutrition Info:

24 g carb, 235 cal, 10 g fat, 3 g sat fat, 29 mg chol, 5 g fib, 10 g pro, 353 mg sod • Carb Choices: 1 1/2; Exchanges: 1 1/2 starch, 1 plant- based protein, 2 fat

Alphabetical Index

W